HERBS TO HELP

Twenty herbal remedies for bestowing the blessing of healthy, refreshing sleep on sufferers from insomnia. Herbal teas and tisanes are not habit-forming, nor do they produce side-effects, unlike the harmful narcotics used to manufacture sleeping pills.

By the same author
FREE FOR ALL
HERBAL TEAS FOR HEALTH AND HEALING
THE HEALING POWER OF HERBAL TEAS

In this series
HERBS AND FRUIT FOR SLIMMERS
HERBS AND FRUIT FOR VITAMINS
HERBS FOR FIRST AID AND MINOR AILMENTS
HERBS FOR HEALTHY HAIR
HERBS FOR INDIGESTION

HERBS TO HELP YOU SLEEP

by
CERES

Drawings by Alison Ross

THORSONS PUBLISHERS LIMITED
Wellingborough, Northamptonshire

First published 1972
Fifth Impression 1984

ISBN 0 7225 0207 9

Printed and bound in Great Britain
by Richard Clay (The Chaucer Press), Ltd.,
Bungay, Suffolk.

CONTENTS

INTRODUCTION

There has been plenty of time to learn about the virtues of herbs, for 'the lore of Herbs', according to Sir Edward Salisbury, the famous botanist, 'may well go back to the time when Stone Age man was the subject of experimentation, both culinary and medicinal, by Stone Age woman'. So at any rate, our presentday knowledge of the use of herbs has thousands of years' experience behind it to show how certain plants can put us right, harmlessly and gently, healthwise.

But hear the other side of the story first. If you have lost the habit of healthy refreshing sleep, you may go to the doctor. Modern orthodox medicine has little to offer except harmful narcotics, most of which originate from the poisonous opium poppy. For sleeplessness, the usual doctors' help seems to be to prescribe drugs in the form of sleeping-pills which are more or less habit-forming according to their make-up, their strength and the character and constitution of the recipient.

The use of these drug-containing sleeping-pills has an anaesthetizing effect on the consciousness and brain, which may outlast the sleeping period. This could well be dangerous, for habitual users lose any accurate self-judgment as to whether they are properly 'awake' or not. 'Beginners', as it were, are aware of heaviness and sleepiness that may last for an increasing amount of time, day after day, after they have woken and got up.

Unfortunately many people find in time that these drugs have less effect and so more are taken, to the great detriment of the taker's well-being. The whole business is frightening and unnecessary.

There are many harmless, even health-giving, non-habit-forming herbs or simples (see *Herbs for First-Aid and Minor Ailments* in this series for a definition of a 'simple') that may help you to sleep. They have no after-effects and it is far wiser to try to find something among those which suits you. You will find pictures and information about twenty of them in this book.

An ordinarily physically and mentally healthy person falls asleep naturally when he goes to bed after a day's work. He goes on sleeping, unless disturbed, for several hours. There is no hard and fast rule as to how many hours everyone needs: some people can do with nine hours regularly, others need only four — the criterion is how long *you* need to refresh *you*.

As everyone knows, sleep is essential for the refreshment of both mind and body. It is the culmination of one day's living and working and the preparation for the next. It may not be so generally known that there are different levels of sleep and that people go through them all several times a night during natural sleep. Scientists have proved now that special levels of sleep are necessary for complete refreshment. Sleeping-pill sleep does not enable you to reach those levels — that is why it is not so refreshing.

Bearing the desire and necessity to re-establish the pattern for natural sleep in mind, let your approach to the problem of your sleeplessness be primarily a common-sense one and try to find out *why* it is that you are not sleeping properly.

If, of course, you suspect that there is something badly wrong with you, for sleeplessness can be a symptom of ill-health, it is important to go to a doctor or qualified medical herbalist. If basically you feel all right, except for very minor ailments, try to think out the reasons why you may be staying awake, or are unable to relax for a good night's sleep.

Don't forget that sleep is a habit. Have you given this habit every chance to work automatically and seen that you are comfortable; not too hot, or too chilly, or that your bed-clothes are not too heavy?

Now that man-made, terylene-filled 'downs' and pillows are cheap, they are better than the old feather-filled types that robbed so many young birds of their parents' nesting down. Those filled with synthetic stuffing are beautifully light *and* washable and they cannot be accused of starting off hay-fever, which the old feather-filled ones were often guilty of, being even worse when they got worn and dusty.

Have you asked yourself if your mattress is firm enough, or does it sag and prevent your spine from getting the support it needs? Many people with and without 'bad backs' have a long, wide board under their mattress and derive much benefit from sleeping straighter and without the continual 'bounce' of a highly sprung mattress against a sprung base.

If you are sure you are comfortable, what else is keeping you awake? Is it air or road traffic noise, or someone's radio or TV, or even someone else snoring? Try one of the soothing herbs and buy some earplugs if so.

Perhaps you are hungry by the time you go to bed if it is a long time since you have eaten. A hot drink often helps, especially a herbal tisane, or tea. Try a cup of Lime-flower or Chamomile tea at bedtime (see p.17). If you've a slight headache your herbalist may recommend a few drops of Alfalfa tincture (see p.13).

If you have a late, heavy meal it may be indigestion that is stopping you from getting off to sleep. Try to cultivate the habit of an early light meal, rather than a late indigestible dinner. The choice of herbs for indigestion is extremely wide and depends, as it does in all medicines that cater for individuals, on your condition and temperament.

Some, like Chamomile, are also helpful for constipation which is a real deterrent to sound sleep.

Primrose tea is recommended for hypersensitive people if they are highly strung and almost uncontrollably restless.

For nervousness, coupled with sleeplessness and fear of storms, thunder and lightning, Rhododendron or 'Snow-rose' is occasionally suggested.

At times of great sorrow and grief, Ignatia or 'St Ignatius' Bean' is invaluable.

Some people are frightened to go to sleep because when they do they have such horrifying nightmares. They can find herbs to help them, like Peony or 'Pentecost Rose'. There is also Heartsease for anyone who has frightening dreams or for those whose limbs jerk about as they are going off to sleep (which sometimes wakes them up again) or who feel that they are whirling round in everlasting vertigo. Spurge Laurel (*Daphne indica*) may help people who dream of terrifying large black cats!

Different herbs, too, soothe different pains that may well be making you sleepless. There is Chamomile for toothache, Valerian and Mullein (*Verbascum*) for earache and Mistletoe for tearing pains in the sciatic nerve, as well as others that you will find in this book.

If, perhaps, you are over-tired, one of the 'cordial' herbs may help you. Many of the best known, sleep-inducing herbs are mild heart tonics or 'cordial' herbs. Heartsease, as its popular name denotes, is one of them, especially if palpitation is another symptom.

On the other hand it may be over-excitement that is keeping you from sleeping, or sheer mental stress. Substitute Maté Tea (made from a South American Oak) for your ordinary Indian or China tea and give up ordinary coffee altogether and drink Dandelion coffee instead. Treat yourself to a Hop pillow (George III gave one to his wife), or slip a few sprigs of Rosemary and a Bay-leaf into your ordinary pillowcase and read about Hops (on p. 22), or Night-flowering Cactus (on p.15).

Do you give yourself every chance for getting into the right mood for sleep? Have a quiet, restful evening, if it is possible, before you go to bed. Although some people like reading thrillers to send them off to sleep, many more are soothed by a few minutes reading from a book that is less exciting, like a book of poems or an anthology about a subject that particularly interests them. Some find familiar, gentle music helpful, but keep it quiet unless you want to keep everyone else awake!

Above all, one of the most important hints to regain a good natural sleeping habit is the need for fresh air. Notice in this book how many herbs help those who are better in fresh air. A walk before bedtime provides a measure of relaxation as well as fresh air. If you cannot go out, open the window wide and do deep breathing exercises, and keep them going while you undress and until you are lying down and thinking happy thoughts of people or places that you love.

Push your worries right away, which is easier than it sounds if you tell yourself that it won't help to toss them around *now*, and that if necessary you'll think of them again in the morning!

Never look at the time, it only makes you more anxious if you do. Give the herbs you are trying a chance to help you and they will. There's no point in doing anything at all but relaxing, and then you will soon be asleep.

Goodnight!!

'Now, blessings light on him that first invented sleep! It covers a man all over, thoughts and all, like a cloak; it is meat for the hungry, drink for the thirsty, heat for the cold and cold for the hot. It is the current coin that purchases all the pleasures of the world cheap, and the balance that sets the king and the shepherd, the fool and the wise man, even.'

Cervantes

NOTE

The dried herbs mentioned in the text can be obtained from health food stores or herbal shops. Unless otherwise stated on the packet, the usual way of making a herbal tea, or infusion, is to pour one pint of boiling water on to one teaspoonful of the herb. A few herbal tinctures such as Alfalfa can also be purchased from health food and herbal shops. Be sure that they have directions with them. If it is essential to sweeten the tea, always use honey instead of sugar.

1
ALFALFA
(*Medicago sativa*)

Alfalfa, or Lucerne, as it is also commonly called, is a green fodder crop for cattle, which can be cut over and over again. Its roots go so deep that ordinary drought does not affect it. It has purple flowers, rather in the form of an elongated, narrow clover-head. It used to be given to cattle as a fattener! Now that everyone wants lean meat, it isn't used as much, although it is still a wonderful general conditioner.

From other points of view, the plant is full of interest. Agricultural botanists have discovered that Alfalfa is one of the plants which show boron deficiency. When boron is not present, Alfalfa's terminal leaves go yellow. Boron is a trace element essential for plant health, of which very little indeed is needed to make the soil healthy for good growth.

Biochemists found too that Alfalfa was a source of Vitamin K, which is the blood-clotting vitamin. It is obvious that this plant still has many unknown virtues.

Although Alfalfa grows on waste ground in this country, it is probably a native of Mediterranean areas for its virtues were highly extolled by Roman writers. Its use is ancient too in Spain, Persia and Peru.

As a medicinal herb (when the whole plant has been used to make tincture) Alfalfa is a good tonic and induces quiet, reposeful and refreshing sleep. It helps headaches and ensures a bright, well feeling on awakening.

One authority said that it dissipates all 'the blues'.

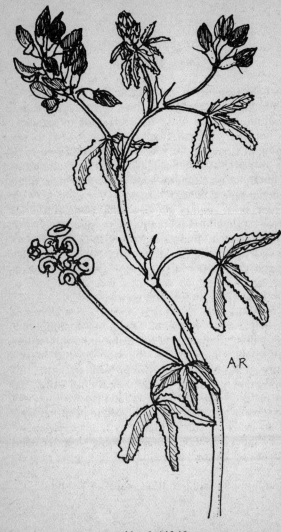

No. 1 Alfalfa

2
CACTUS or NIGHT-FLOWERING CEREUS
(*Cactus grandiflorus*)

'It is called the Queen of the Night. The flowers open in the evening at sunset and by the next morning they are faded and dead. But like many short-lived flowers, they are some of the finest of all the floral world.' So the horticultural writer, Patrick Synge, says. 'They gleam like great trumpets of light in the darkness, when the owl hoots and the old church clock strikes midnight.'

This queen of the cacti grows and blooms in South America, in Mexico and in the West Indies, where it is also called 'Vanilla Cactus' and 'Sweet-scented Cactus', and its enormous flowers can measure up to three feet in circumference. The inside of the petals is a brilliant yellow and the white centre is filled with a shag of stamens.

Herbalists use the dried, fragrant flowers to make a tea to help those who are sleepless and who feel as if their bodies are in a cage because of an iron band round their hearts or bladders or other parts. It is also good for those who are sad and melancholy, who fear death and who are frightened by feeling the pulsating of their own hearts. Night-flowering Cereus will help those whose dreams are terrifying and who wake with icy-cold hands, especially if they feel better, ordinarily, when they are in the open air.

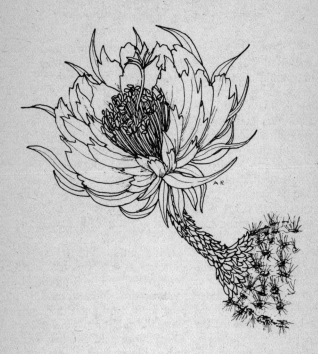

No. 2 Cactus or Night-Flowering Cereus

3
CHAMOMILE
(*Matricaria chamomilla* and *Anthemis nobilis*)

There are two Chamomiles used by herbalists. The first is German Chamomile (*Matricaria chamomilla*), also called 'Bitter Chamomile' or 'Hippocrates' Chamomile', and the second is the 'English, Roman, Common or Belgian' Chamomile (*Anthemis nobilis*).

Both are digestives and soothing, tranquillizing herbs which will help sleeplessness. The first, German Chamomile, is useful for people who are restless, peevish, constipated or who have earache or ringing in the ears, or toothache and who moan and groan a lot when they are asleep and have frightening dreams.

The second, Roman Chamomile, is used for most of the same symptoms, but also for those who are sensitive to cold air and yet have a tickly cough in a warm room and hot, itchy soles to their feet. It is also used when there is a tendency towards frequent urination, or 'frequency' as it can be popularly called.

It was Culpeper who said that 'The bathing with a decoction of chamomile taketh away the weariness, and easeth pain.' He evidently enjoyed 'the flowers boiled in posset drink' when they 'helpeth to expel colds and aches and pains'.

Chamomile lawns were popular long before our familiar grass lawns, one explanation being that until the mid-nineteenth century, grass seed was difficult to get. It is thought that Drake was in all probability playing bowls on a Chamomile lawn on Plymouth Hoe, when the Spanish Armada was sighted.

'Beautiful Chamomile', according to the Elizabethan poet Spenser, 'the more it is trodden on, the better it grows'.

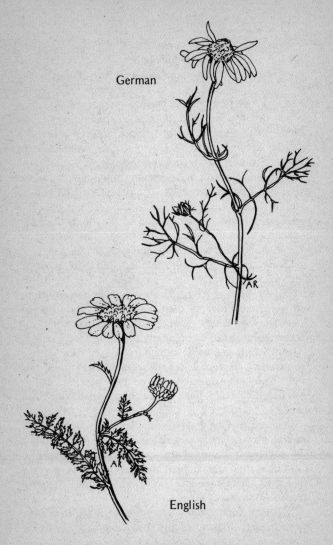

German

English

No. 3 Chamomile

4
COWSLIP
(*Primula veris*)

Milton's charming poem,

> Thus I set my printless feet,
> O'er the Cowslips' velvet head,
> That bends not as I tread.

makes one think of the days when Cowslips were thick and plentiful in chalk and limestone and other meadows. When 'tistie-tostie balls' were made by children who picked off the deliciously scented heads of flowers and then threaded them into tightly packed balls, which were tossed from child to child. There were masses of Cowslips in the fields then. Now they are quite scarce, for so many of their fields have been ploughed up or built over.

Cowslips are also called 'St Peter's Keys', 'Paigles', 'Palsywort' and 'Gaskins'. Indeed, their country names are endless, which shows how everyone knew and loved them. Even Shakespeare mentions them in his fairy play *A Midsummer Night's Dream*.

> Where the bee lurks, there lurk I
> In a Cowslip's bell I lie.

The flowers have long been used for candying, for salads and for wine-making, and Coleridge said of Cowslip wine that:

> It is a wine of virtuous powers
> My mother made it of wild flowers.

Wine, by the way, used to be used as a soother of nerves and other ailments as well as an intoxicating drink.

Cowslip tea, and occasionally a few drops of Cowslip tincture, is used medicinally by herbalists to give quiet sleep if taken before going to bed. Different authorities say that it is good for cramp, vertigo, buzzing in the ears, especially if the skin on the forehead is tense, and to ease the sensation of a band round the head. Cowslip tea or tincture is to help those who always feel better in the fresh air.

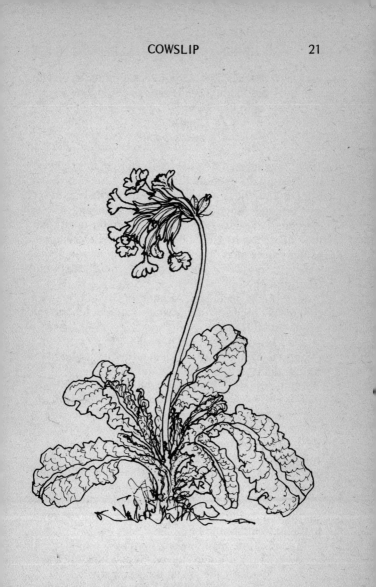

No. 4 Cowslip

5
HOPS
(*Humulus lupulus*)

There have apparently always been Hops in this country, for botanists are convinced that they are natives of Britain. They have not, however, always been used for beer-making, although once they were in general use, everyone was agreed, except John Evelyn the diarist that they made the best beer that England has ever known. Evelyn wrote that 'Hops have transmuted our wholesome ale into *beer*, which doubtless much alters our constitutions.'

Many herbs, including 'Alehoof' or Ground Ivy, were commonly used in the making of ale before the popularity of Hops.

> Hops, reformation, bays and beer
> Came into England all in one year.

runs an old saying, and the year was 1524.

Hopfields are a common sight in various districts, especially in Kent where they are cultivated extensively and where oast houses for their drying are a feature of the landscape. The hops' stems grow up the intricately tight strings between their poles, always climbing and winding in a clockwise direction. It is the female 'cones' or 'strobiles', full of strong scent and pollen, that are picked to be used.

There is a pleasing verse of instruction to hop-growers by the old countryman Thomas Tusser, who was living in the sixteenth century:

> Get into thy hop-yard, for now it is time
> To teach Robin Hop on his pole how to clime:
> To follow the sunne, as his property is,
> And weed him and trim him if aught go amiss.

Hops have a variety of country names, including

'Goldings', 'Whitebines', 'Seeders' and 'Colegates'. They are supposed to symbolize injustice!

Hop pillows are much recommended for those who are sleepless, though the smell is rather overpowering. Hop tea used to be sold to be mixed with ordinary tea and herbalists still give it to poor sleepers who also suffer from dizziness, nausea and headaches. It is said to help 'unstrung conditions of the nervous system' and giddiness and stupidity, and anyone who suffers from twitching muscles.

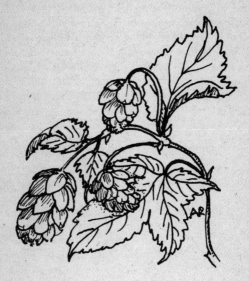

No. 5 Hops

JAMAICA DOGWOOD
(*Piscidia erythrina*)

This tree is common in Jamaica where it fulfils many purposes including the use of its timber and the curious method that the natives have, or had, of employing the juices from its bark and roots to help catch fish! This was done by using a strong decoction which was cast into the water to intoxicate fish so that they rose, floating, to the surface and from thence could easily be netted.

It is a method that has had parallels in other countries, where different herbs were used. Needless to say, the fish were not harmed, except the smallest and weakest which died under the intoxicating anaesthetic; the others recovered consciousness once they had been captured.

The Jamaica Dogwood does not grow in this country except possibly in botanic gardens, but herbalists import it for several proper reasons. A 'boiling' or a decoction, of a small quantity of the bark is a highly astringent solution and of much use in the treatment of internal ulcers; it is also a cure for mange in dogs and herbalists find it invaluable as a sedative for humans. It is very similar in action to, but without the harmful narcotic properties of, Opium, when carefully administered in *small* doses, but it should not be taken unless prescribed by a qualified medical herbalist.

As a herb to help sleeplessness, it can therefore be invaluable if the symptoms merit it being prescribed. It is *not* a herb to prescribe for yourself.

Insomnia due to worry is often vastly helped by it, especially if the sufferer is also troubled by nervous excitement.

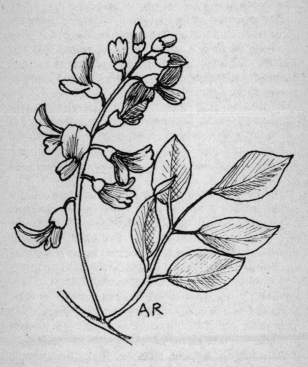

No. 6 Jamaica Dogwood

LADY'S SLIPPER ORCHID
(*Cypripaedium pubescens*)

Lady Rockley, in her book on the wild flowers of the Dominions, wrote,

> The ground orchids are one of Canada's attractions. Particularly the Lady's Slippers or Mocassin-flowers which are almost tropical in effect, in the cold wild spots where they occur. The showy Lady's Slipper is found in Newfoundland and the Eastern Provinces. The flower is large, over two inches across and the petals are white and the pouched lip, which forms the 'slipper' is much inflated and is white and beautifully marked with crimson. To add to its charm the flower is fragrant.

She did not mention its medicinal properties, although they have been known for hundreds of years.

The plant was apparently introduced into the official American *Materia Medica* by Professor Rafinesque, who was once Professor of Medical Botany in the University of Transylvania. He said:

> I am able to introduce for the first time this beautiful genus into our Materia Medica; all species are equally remediable, they have long been known to the Indians, who called them 'Mocassin-flowers' and were used by the empyrics of New England ... They produce beneficial effects in all nervous diseases and hysterical affections by allaying pain, quietening the nerves and promoting sleep and have no baneful or narcotic effect.

As a sleep-inducer a mild infusion or tea of Lady's Slipper Orchid, 'Mocassin-Flower' 'Noah's Ark' or 'American Valerian', may be recommended by herbalists, especially for those who suffer from over-stimulation of the brain, including children who cry out or start laughing and wanting to play in the night.

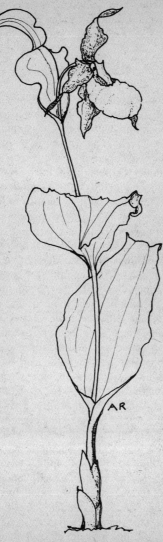

No. 7 Lady's Slipper Orchid

LAVENDER
(*Lavendula vera*)

Everyone knows Lavender. It is possibly our best-loved garden herb. It is notable for its delicious smell and its delightful association with bees and summer and sunshine, and looks lovely as a single bush, or as a hedge as a backing for brighter coloured flowers.

Dried Lavender flowers keep their scent for years, and Parkinson in his old herbal *Paradisus* was quite correct when he described its fragrance as 'piercing the senses'.

The early settlers took Lavender and many other familiar garden herbs and simples with them when they set out for the New World. It was sad that they found Lavender died and they couldn't propagate it, and so came to the conclusion that 'it is not for this Climate'.

At home Lavender has been used for 'the vapours, the migraines and other little remedies' for countless generations, probably since it was brought to this country by the Romans. In fact it was the Romans who found that a Lavender bath is very soothing to an over-active brain.

For simple, uncomplicated, sporadic sleeplessness, try a Lavender bath (see p. 54 for instructions for a Rosemary bath and follow those), and then sprinkle a few drops of strong essence of Lavender or a good Lavender perfume on your pillow. The effort of breathing in the delicious scent, with deep, regular breaths, often has the desired effect of sending you off to sleep!

In *The Garden of Health* which William Langham wrote nearly 400 years ago, he gave this enchanting advice for the use of Lavender: 'Smell it often to comfort and cleare the sight. Boyle it in water and wett thy shirt in it and dry it again and weare it.' He goes on

to add, 'Shread the herbe with the flowers and distill it
and drink two ounces of the water to help the giddiness
of the head and rub the head all over with it and let it
dry in by itselfe.'

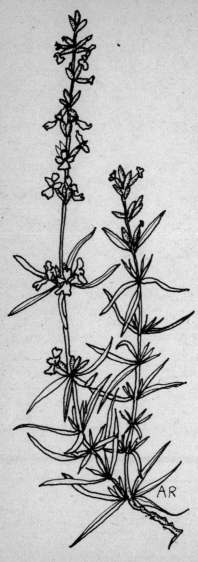

No. 8 Lavender

LETTUCE
(*Lactuca virosa*)

This Lettuce is a wild species. In appearance it is nothing like the leaf-tight globes and ovals that we grow in our gardens for salads.

Botanists are not even sure that *Lactuca virosa* which is a common weed, is a wild native of Britain, although it turns up by roadsides and on waste places very frequently. It can often be found on disturbed ground, and many plants appeared on bombed sites during and after the Second World War, even in the hearts of cities.

It is a tall (six feet or over) plant and has small, pale yellow flowers and long, thin, pale green, oval leaves.

Its reputation as a harmless herb to help encourage sleep is very old. Even its country names show that, for it has been called 'Sleep-wort' ('wort' meaning weed or herb in the old days) since Anglo-Saxon times. It was also known as 'Lettuce Opium', although it has nothing to do with real opium.

The stems and leaves of this plant, as well as those of other lettuces, exude white juice when they are broken, and the Chinese used to make their 'sleeping-milk' or *Ku-chin-kan* from this.

Before the days of anaesthetics, 'soporific sponges' were employed to give a measure of relief from conscious agony, and this particular wild lettuce juice was used, with other plant juices, on these sponges.

Medicinally, wild or 'acrid' Lettuce acts on the circulatory system and the brain. Wild Lettuce tea is a useful herbal sedative, especially for those who have a tickling cough, are restless and have cramp in the legs, and who find it impossible to get to sleep because of all or any of these reasons.

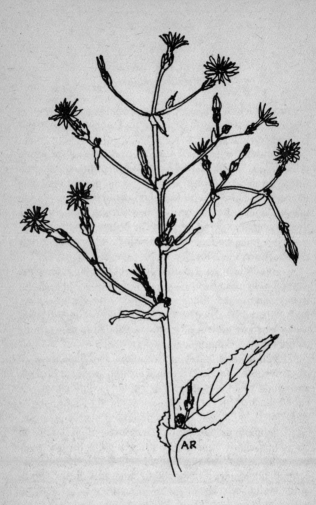

No. 9 Lettuce

LILY OF THE VALLEY
(*Convallaria majallis*)

According to Gerard, the seventeenth-century herbalist, Lilies of the valley used to grow abundantly very near London on 'Hampsted Heath and Bushie Heath'. Now they grow in a rampageous, naturalized fashion in a few woods only, the nearest being perhaps within forty miles of the city. There is nothing lovelier to find than a bed of these 'May Lilies', or *Muguets*, as the French call them, or even 'Lilies-among-Thorns', or 'Our Lady's Tears' as they used to be called in this country. They are such an outstanding wild flower, there is no wonder that they are surrounded by superstition and myth.

One old story says that their scent draws the nightingale to choose his mate in the deepest dell in the wood; and another, that they only grow wild where the blood of a good man or a saint has fallen.

Be that as it may, Lilies of the valley have therapeutic values apart from the aesthetic delights they give by their charming appearance and scent. Abraham Cowley made the somewhat ambiguous statement that 'No plant kinder to the brain doth live'. The plant is known to have been used as a cordial herb and mild heart tonic for centuries.

Lily of the valley used under the direction of a medical herbalist can induce quiet sleep in which there will be no horrifying dreams or nightmares. It is a useful soother for the irritable, it overcomes depression, and is good for those who suffer from palpitation at night or who feel that their hearts suddenly stop and then start again. It is credited with power to help those that grate their teeth in their sleep. It is another herb for anyone who feels better in the open air.

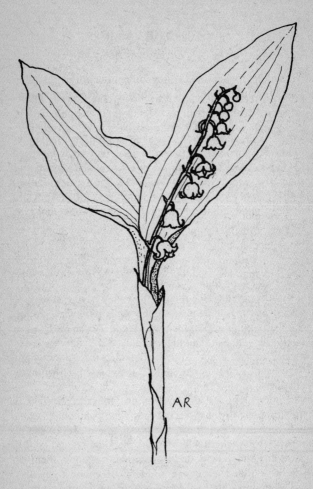

No. 10 Lily of the Valley

11
LIME
(*Tilia europaea*)

Lime trees are often planted by local authorities in urban streets and what could be lovelier, except for the officials' terrible habit of having them lopped back so hard each winter, that the poor trees have nothing but a tight green mop of leaves and can never flower.

A naturally developed Lime tree, in full leaf, is a graceful and beautiful shape, often having 'petticoats' round its base where twigs and shoots have developed like a small reflection of its rounded crown. In flower, in late June or early July, the scent from the flowers can be almost overpowering in humid weather, and bees and other nectar-gatherers all enjoy the brief harvest.

It is the flowers with their curious bracts that are used to make the famous tea or tisane, *tilleul*, which is a mild, honey-scented drink that is soothing and delicious. It is an excellent nerve tonic and very good for relieving the stuffed-up feeling of colds. Oddly enough it has a strengthening effect on the muscles of the eyes and is generally very purifying to the blood.

As a herb to help the sleepless, lime-flower tea can be splendid for those who start to sweat soon after falling asleep or those who have any mild neuralgias.

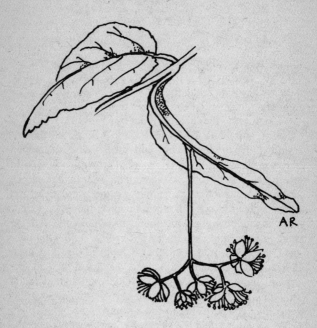

No. 11 Lime

12
OATS
(*Avena sativa*)

This wild oat is a menace to farmers. Its seed can lie in the earth for years, waiting for the right conditions for germination, and when it does come up there is only one way of getting rid of it and that is to pull it out by hand. In huge fields such as there are on the Cotswolds, this becomes an enormous task. But the strength and the virility of the plant are shown by its ability to go on appearing when farmers and growers have been trying to eradicate it for so long.

There are many varieties and forms of cultivated oat and over fifty different species of other wild oats all over the world, in the temperate regions of both hemispheres.

Oats are good food for the brain and tradition has it that it is porridge made from oats that has made the Scots into such a fine, hard-working race.

Medicinally, for no specified reason whatsoever, wild oats appear to be one of the herbs that help women more than men! Oats can make a fine tonic after debilitating diseases and help nervous exhaustion and strengthen the ability to keep the mind on one subject at a time. A few drops of the fluid extract, or tincture, or a tea, may help those who are unable to sleep, especially if they are suffering from a mild headache with catarrhal disorders as well.

Meredith, in a few words, created a lovely image of fields of crops when he wrote: 'Yellow oats and brown wheat and barley, pale as rye.'

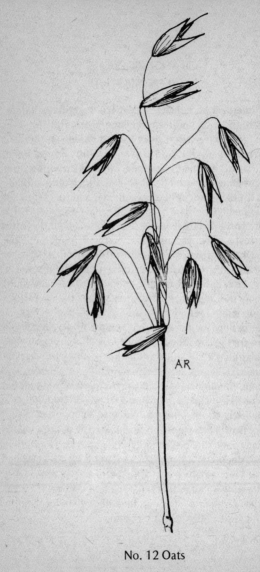

No. 12 Oats

ORANGE BUDS
(*Citrus aurantium*)

Oranges were the 'golden apples' of legendary fame. They were first brought to England from Italy in the fifteenth and sixteenth centuries and have been cultivated here since 1595, in stove houses. There were actually 'some great Orange trees' out in the open in a garden in Beddington in Surrey, which John Evelyn knew well (so we can read in his Diary), and he regretted that they were killed by the great frost in 1739-40.

Others grew in gardens at Salcombe in Devon, 'one of the warmest places in the British Isles'. The pleasure of growing Orange trees in this country increased and really popularized the idea of having a heated greenhouse or orangery. Orangeries were at the height of their fame in Britain in the seventeenth and eighteenth centuries. According to a French book of that period, *Histoire Naturelle des Orangiers*, by Risso, 169 different kinds of oranges were in cultivation then.

No one seems to know how the wearing of orange blossom became associated with brides. The flowers are pure white, smell delicious and look perfect with their parchment-like perianth segments, so all those attributes would be excuse enough.

These flowers may be used medicinally, especially when they are in bud, by those who suffer from disturbed sleep, or from much incontrollable yawning when they are awake, or from right-sided neuralgia of the face and from headaches, nausea and vertigo. Orange bud tea is available from a few herbalists or health stores, but it can be difficult to obtain.

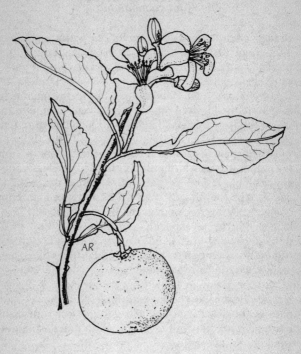

No. 13 Orange Buds

PASQUE FLOWER
(*Anemone pulsatilla*)

How strange it is that among the herbs to help you sleep are two of our loveliest flowers, Lilies of the valley and Pasque Flowers, or *Pulsatilla* as they are usually known to herbalists and homoeopaths.

Pasque flowers, or 'Easter Flowers', 'Meadow Blue Anemones' or 'Wind Flowers' are very uncommon wild flowers but are still found in rough grass on a few hillsides in Gloucestershire, Hertfordshire, Cambridgeshire and Suffolk.

They have been cultivated in gardens for over 400 years, having originally, it is thought, been lifted from wild stock which was thus depleted. In gardens they are nothing like as beautiful as they can look on a wild, sunny slope.

This plant has a long history of curative powers. Culpeper mentions its ability to help many complaints from 'the leprosy', to 'the leaves being stamped and the juice sniffed up the nose, [when it] purgeth the head mightily. So doth the root being chewed in the mouth.' There is, however, no need for such drastic action when the Pasque Flower is used as a mild sedative. When it is prescribed, provided always that the sufferer's symptoms tally with those that the plant is said to cure, it can prove highly efficacious.

The symptoms to encourage the use of *Pulsatilla* are that it helps those who like lying with their hands above their heads and who must have several pillows. It is for sensitive people, especially women, who fear the dark and ghosts! It helps to soothe children who like to be fussed and anyone who has a dry mouth, without thirst, or who is wide awake when they go to bed after being sleepy all the afternoon and early evening. It appears to be indicated again for those that love fresh air and being out of doors and whose legs feel tired and heavy when they get to bed.

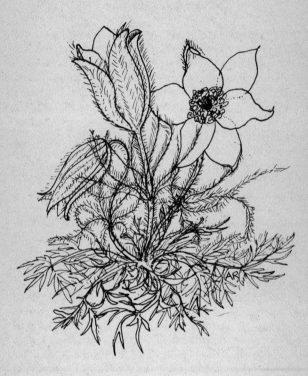

No. 14 Pasque Flower

15
PASSION-FLOWER
(*Passiflora incarnata*)

There are many different species of Passion-flower. In Britain, the blue Passion-flower *Passiflora caerulea* (see picture on page 47) will grow and flower and sometimes fruit out of doors, but it is tender and cannot stand frost. The Edible Passion-flower (*P. edulis*) is cultivated too, but in greenhouses where it will produce large, deep purple fruits which are delicious and exotic in flavour when added to a fruit salad, their jelly-like seeds giving the whole an unusual fragrance and flavour.

The Passion-flower that is used herbally, as a sedative, is *Passiflora incarnata* or the Rosy Passion-flower, and it grows in warm parts of America and in the West Indies. It is said to have orange-coloured 'apple-sized' fruits which, according to Johnson's edition of Gerard's *Herbal*, were called 'Granadillas' by the Spaniards in the West Indies and 'Maracoe' by the Virginians. In America, it appears that they are known as 'May-bobs' or 'May-apples'.

The *Passiflora* genus was so named because the floral arrangements of many of the Passion-flowers were supposed by Spanish friars to represent 'the Passion of our Saviour'. The three stigmas in the centre were said to look like the three nails; the five anthers, the five wounds. The corona stood for the crown of thorns, or the halo of glory; and the ten sepals, the apostles, without Judas and Peter. The sharp whip-like tendrils represented the scourges of His persecutors.

On the recommendation of a qualified herbalist, Passion-flower tea produces good refreshing sleep for those who are restless and wakeful after exhaustion or are mentally worried and overworked. It can also help a night cough.

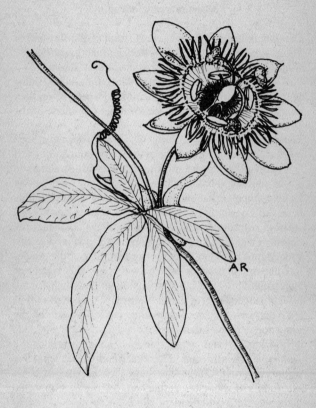

No. 15 Passion-Flower

16
RED CLOVER
(*Trifolium pratense var. sativum*)

There is nothing lovelier in high summer than a field of flowering Red Clover with bees enjoying its heavily scented heads and with butterflies all round it too.

Clouded Yellow butterflies love it, and as they come only sparsely to Britain during hot summers, when they overflow, as it were, from the Continent, it is one of the best places to look out for them.

Red Clover is a native of Britain but has been cultivated and carefully selected to produce the best forage crops for cattle. It is often sown with Rye grass to give a nourishing hay or silage crop.

The popular names for Red Clover, which include such old favourites as 'Cow-grass' or 'Tinker-tailor' grass (though, of course, it is not a grass at all) show that the countryman associated this plant with grazing animals. Indeed the world 'Clover' was derived from the Anglo-Saxon word *Cloefre* which was also the name of Hercules' club. The club on our playing cards is named after the Clover trefoil or three-leafletted leaves. It is also the sign of the Shamrock, 'St Patrick's Herb', by which he demonstrated the Trinity.

Medicinally the plant contains useful minerals, and Dr Fernie has said that 'The likelihood is that whatever virtue the Red Clover can boast for counter-acting a scrofulous disposition resides in its highly-elaborated lime, silica and other earthy salts.'

Herbalists use it to help sleeplessness for those who have a bad cough which is worse at night, and those who suffer from cold hands and feet; or from a poor memory and who are confused and have a headache when they do wake.

'Clover blossoms, or honey-suckers, as some call them, should be gathered in when the dew is on them', according to an old settler's notebook in the U.S.A.

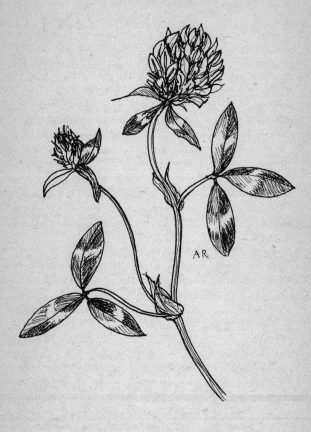

No. 16 Red Clover

17

RED POPPY
(*Papaver rhoeas*)

Although the Opium Poppy is so poisonous and has been the source of so many drugs, like opium, morphine, laudanum and codein, the Red Poppy, or the 'Flanders Poppy', is harmless and a useful soporific when properly prescribed.

It used to be a familiar sight in cornfields. Now selective weed-killers and careful screening of the corn grain have to a great extent exterminated it in all but a few remote areas. However, a few of these beautiful 'Corn-roses' can still be seen in odd field corners and on waste ground and beside unsprayed roadsides.

It has several country names, one of which is 'Bleedwort' and another is 'Headaches'. Some poet has suggested that:

> Corn poppies that in crimson dwell,
> Called headaches from their sickly smell.

But to contradict this comes an old herbal hint:

For a sick headache

Make and drink a tea of Poppy Flowers and Saffron, then go to bed, be very still and do not have a noise.

Possibly the verse is sheer poet's license, because there is no mention of any scent at all, let alone a sickly one, by botanists from these gay flowers. Red Poppy seeds are used on bread and in soups sometimes, for sedative purposes.

> That Ceres with my flow'r is grieved
> Some think, but they are much deceived
> For where her richest Corn she sows
> The inmate Poppy she allows
> Together both our seed doth fling
> And bids us both together spring;

Good, 'cause my sleep-giving juice
Does more than Corn to life induce.
                            Abraham Cowley

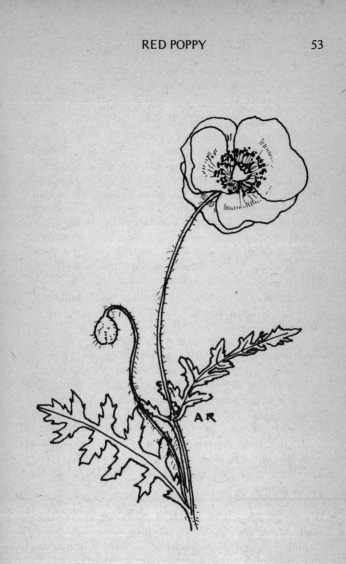

No. 17 Red Poppy

18

ROSEMARY
(*Rosmarinus officinalis*)

'There's Rosemary, that's for remembrance.' Shakespeare said. It is also one of the most soothing, sleep-inducing herbs we have, and a delightful shrub to have in the garden, for its blue flowers are out all through the winter. It is one of the herbs with so many different actions, internally and externally. In the latter way it is stimulating to some people, so the essence, which is easily prepared for a bath by boiling a good handful of the tips of the young branches for about ten minutes, should not be used too close to bedtime.

Rosemary can be dried and kept in a tightly lidded jar for years without losing its smell. A few sprigs of it slipped inside the pillow-case, with a Bayleaf, as suggested in the Introduction, make a lovely fragrant pillow which, however, does need refreshing frequently.

> Rosemary is bothe tree and heerbe ... It tempreth, comforteth and savth the brayne and all the heede ... also the leves layde under the heede — whanne a man slepes — it letteth and doeth away with evell spirits and varytees of the night and suffreth not to dreeme fowle dreemes nor to be aferde. But he must be out of deedely synne for it is an holy tree.

Thus wrote a sixteenth-century herbalist, Richard Banckes.

Rosemary is much associated with Christmas and the custom of bringing in the boar's head, which may have originated at Queen's College, Oxford.

Medicinally it is known to be soothing to the nerves and to help those who are wakeful to go peacefully to sleep, especially if they suffer from icy coldness of the feet.

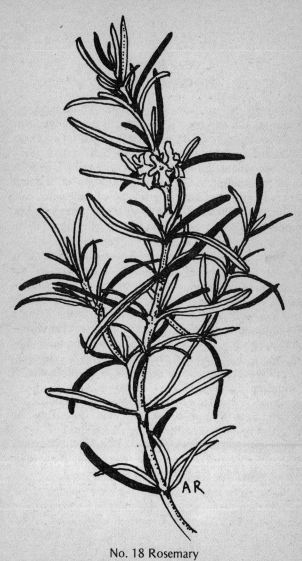

No. 18 Rosemary

19

SCULLCAP
(*Scutellaria lateritiflora*)

This herb is an American species of Scullcap, or Skullcap, as many people spell it. It is one of the finest nerve-soothing herbs known, and has been used to cure hydrophobia since the eighteenth-century.

Modern herbalists use it for nervous patients and for those who suffer a lot from nausea, hiccough, stomach pain and migraine, especially for those whose worst pain is over the right eye. It is also very conducive to quiet, gentle sleep-giving, and helps anyone who has a fear of calamity, sudden wakefulness and night terrors.

There are two Scullcaps in Britain, one (*Scutellaria minor*) a small, pink-flowered, bog-loving plant and the other (*S. galericulata*) a waterside beauty with pairs of bright cobalt hooded flowers. One of its country names is 'Hoodwort' and a writer on natural history, Alison Ross, has given a picture of it, as it grows: 'Hoodwort, growing by a stream, among green rushes and sedges and spear-long Iris leaves is eye-catching only to the most carefully searching wild-flowerer by virtue of its pairs of twin deep blue flowers.'

Dried Scullcap, for making a herbal tea, if bought at a health store or from a herbalist, must be kept in an air-tight jar with a tightly screwed-down lid or it will deteriorate and become useless.

It is sometimes used as a compound herb, with Valerian or other simples.

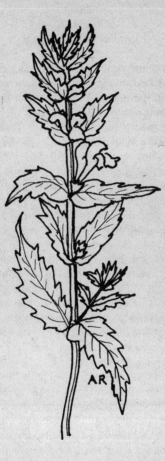

No. 19 Scullcap

20

VALERIAN
(*Valeriana officinalis*)

Valerian has a very good, very ancient reputation and must be one of our most popular wild herbs. Certainly if popularity can be judged by the number of its country names, it would come near to the top of the list. Here are a few of them: 'Setwell', 'Capon's Taile', 'All-heal' (see *Herbs for First-aid and Minor Ailments* for more about 'All-heals' and 'Self-heals'), and 'Swetall'. Its funniest country name is 'Phu' — but its flower smell is really too pleasant to warrant such an expression of disgust, and 'Phu' may have described its crushed roots.

But it is its scent, or the scent of the crushed root, that cats and other animals adore. Some people suggest that Valerian juice was smeared on to the person of the Pied Piper to attract cats and rats, though the latter would surely have attracted the former, without needing Valerian too!

Valerian may have been one of the ingredients of St Mary Magdalene's lovely soothing ointment. At any rate it is known as a 'Blessed Herb'. It used to be, and still may be, grown specially in Derbyshire, where the 'Valerie growers' were famous.

As a sleep-inducing herb, taken carefully and only on the prescription of a qualified herbalist as it is dangerous to mix it with orthodox drugs, it is helpful for over-sensitive people and for those who have the sensation in bed, just before going to sleep, that they are floating in the air. It also helps those who are irritable or tremulous and who have pressure in their foreheads or a cold head. It is useful for earache from draughts and cold and for those who may start choking on falling asleep.

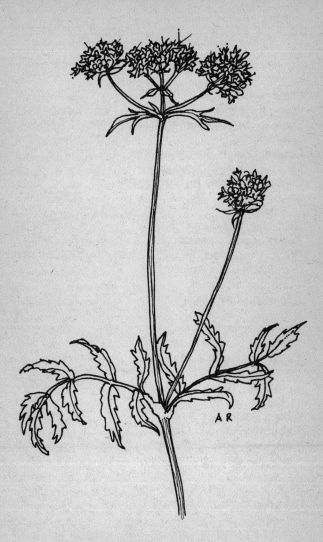

No. 20 Valerian

THERAPEUTIC INDEX

Blood purifier, Lime
'Blues, the', Alfalfa
Brain, over-stimulation of, Lady's Slipper Orchid, Lavender
Catarrh, Oats
Choking, Valerian
Cold air, sensitivity to, Chamomile
Cold feet, head, hands, Cactus, Red Clover, Rosemary, Valerian
Confusion, Red Clover
Constipation, Chamomile
Cough, Chamomile, Lettuce, Passion-flower, Red Clover
Cramp, Cowslip, Lettuce
Death, fear of, Cactus
Depression, Lily of the Valley
Dizziness, Hops
Dreams, see Nightmares
Dry mouth, Pasque Flower
Earache, Chamomile, Mullein p.10), Valerian
Ears, ringing or buzzing in, Chamomile, Cowslip
Excitement, Bay p. 10, Cactus, Hops, Jamaica Dogwood, Maté p. 10, Rosemary
Exhaustion, Passion-flower
Exhaustion, nervous, Oats
Eyes, Lime, Scullcap
Fears (of dark, ghosts, etc.), Cactus, Pasque Flower, Scullcap
Feet, itching soles of, Chamomile
'Floating in the air', Valerian
'Frequency', Chamomile
Fresh air (better in), p. 11, Cactus, Cowslip, Lily of the Valley, Pasque Flower

Ulcers, internal, Jamaica Dogwood
Urination, frequent, Chamomile
Vertigo, Cowslip, Heartsease p. 10, Orange Buds
Wakefulness, Pasque Flowers, Passion-flower, Rosemary,
   Scullcap
Worry, Jamaica Dogwood
Yawning, Orange Buds